The
SENIOR CITIZENS'
SURVIVAL GUIDE

BEYOND THE NEW MILLENNIUM

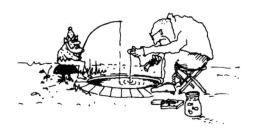

The

SENIOR CITIZENS' SURVIVAL GUIDE

BEYOND THE NEW MILLENNIUM

Bob Feigel

and

Malcolm Walker

CCC Publications

Chatsworth, California

Published by

CCC Publications
9725 Lurline Avenue
Chatsworth, CA 91311

U.S. Copyright ©1999 Bob Siegel & Malcolm Walker

Published by arrangement with Saint Publishing Ltd. of Auckland, New Zealand;
(©1996 Bob Siegel & Malcolm Walker)

U.S. version manufactured in the United States of America

Cover ©1999 CCC Publications

Interior text & illustrations ©1999 CCC Publications

Cover production by Klaus Selbrede

ISBN: 1-57644-083-4

If your local U.S. bookstore is out of stock, copies of this book may be obtained by mailing check or money order for $6.95 per book (plus $3.00 to cover postage and handling) to: CCC Publications; 9725 Lurline Avenue, Chatsworth, CA 91311

Pre-publication Edition – 1/99

Senior Citizen: (lsi:nje lsitzen) adj.,n
Anyone aged 55 and over who still thinks life is worth living.

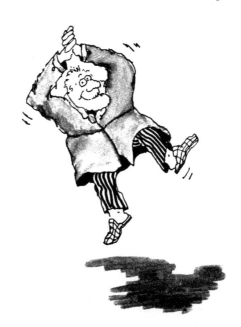

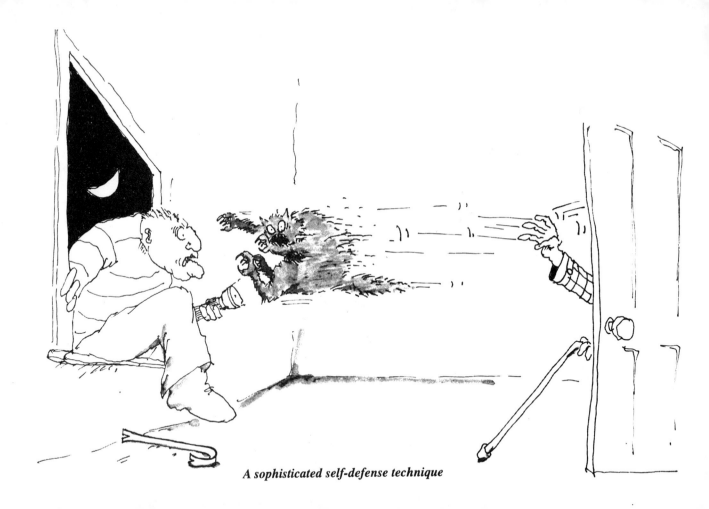

A sophisticated self-defense technique

INTRODUCTION

The Senior Citizen
In enlightened societies, Senior Citizens are venerated.
They are placed high upon pedestals of honor and respect.
They are listened to by their children and by their children's children. Each word, each opinion cherished as priceless pearls of wisdom.
Senior Citizens are treasured in their Golden Years. Pampered through the Autumn of their lives. Not only that, but their wishes are carried out before they are!
In enlightened societies, the older you get, the better IT gets.
Unfortunately, unless you understand 中文 and eat with chopsticks, you can forget it.

A Raw Deal
So what's it like being a Senior Citizen in today's unenlightened western society?
How about bleak?
After all, you've spent a lifetime working, paying taxes, playing by the rules. And now, just when your investment should start paying dividends, you're tossed out ... banished. Exiled to geriatric ghettos for the gray.
Suddenly, no one is listening. Years of experience mean nothing. Your opinions don't count. You've been sentenced to an almost ghost-like existence on the sidelines of a society that thinks nothing of milking you for every last cent you've got.
No doubt about it — you're getting a raw deal.

Fighting Back
Then why not retaliate? Get even? Fight back and change this rotten, superficial, youth-oriented culture and transform it into an enlightened society where you don't have to eat with chopsticks.
But first you have to survive and this little handbook can help you do it.

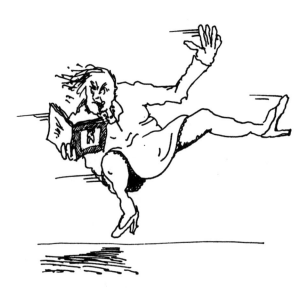

PART I - SWEET BIRD OF YOUTH

GOING ... GOING ... *GONE*!

Introduction

The Warning Signs

It's Too Late When ...

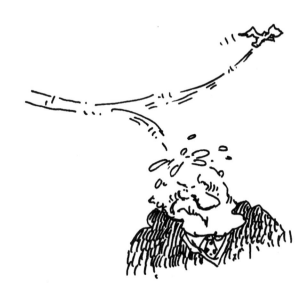

GOING ... GOING ... *GONE*!

Leon Trotsky believed that Old Age was '*the most unexpected of all things that happen to a man.*' Not that he had much time to enjoy his surprise, having unexpectedly met the wrong end of an assassin's ice-pick at the tender age of 61.

Even more to the point, it is often said that '*Youth is a disease from which we all recover.*'

So what are the omens that signal this miraculous metamorphosis? How do we recognize those inexorable harbingers that herald the magic moment when the jaded grub of youth emerges from its dissipated chrysalis of middle age to soar like an eagle upon the golden winds of Autumn?

To put it another way, how do we know if we're already 'over the hill' or simply teetering at the summit of that slippery slide to oblivion?

Let's look at some of the tell-tale signs.

The Warning Signs

You start saying things like: 'In my day ... When I was young ... In the good old days ...'

You can't see the numbers on the bathroom scale without holding your stomach in.

Your doctor starts saying things like: 'Considering your age ...'

The gleam in your eyes is the sun hitting your bifocals.

Your back goes out more than you do.

You find the glasses you've been looking for on your head.

You can't stand intolerant people.

The candles on your birthday cake trigger the smoke alarm.

Your golf score is twice your age.

The thought of exercise makes you sweat.

You feel younger at the class reunion than anyone looks.

You call your wrinkles 'laugh lines'.

You can't stand toilet paper hung in the 'wrong' direction.

You finally decide to procrastinate but never get around to it.

You have to rely on the grandchildren to program your video.

A successful session in the bathroom is one of the highlights of your day.

You realize that the only way to look thinner is to hang around someone fatter.

You can't name one single Top-40 song and wouldn't like any of them anyway.

You feel like the night before, but you haven't been anywhere.

You wake up at three in the morning and spend the rest of the night trying to figure out why.

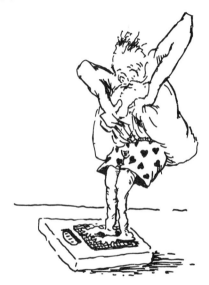

It's Too Late When ...

... being young at heart doesn't change the fact that you're old everywhere else.

... a dripping faucet causes an uncontrollable urge in your bladder.

... your birthday cake collapses from the weight of the candles.

... now that you know the answers, no one asks the questions.

... your hair turns white from worrying about the gray hairs.

... your mind begins to wander and forgets to come back.

... everything hurts and what doesn't hurt doesn't work.

... you sit in a rocking chair and can't make it go.

... you get winded playing bridge.

... your knees buckle but your belt won't.

... you still refer to the refrigerator as an 'ice-box'.

... your mind makes commitments your body can't meet.

... you sink your teeth into a good steak and they stay there.

... your only exercise is as a pallbearer for friends who did exercise.

... a successful session in the bathroom is the *only* highlight of your day.

... the most expensive items at the antique shop are younger than you are.

... you keep an extra pair of glasses to find the other pairs and lose all of them ...

PART II - SURVIVAL SKILLS

SHOPLIFTING FOR BEGINNERS
Introduction
Basic Rules
Child In Stroller Ruse

CREATIVE COOKING WITH PET FOODS
Introduction
You Are What You Eat
Memorable Meals
Our Chef Suggests ...
Sample Recipe
Entertaining For The Impoverished

STAYING HEALTHY
WHILE YOU'RE FALLING APART
Introduction
Exercise Rules
Safe Sex for Seniors
Personal Spa Bath

GLAMOUR FOR GERIATRICS
Introduction
Do-It-Yourself Face-Lifts
Staying In Style
Salvation Army Fashion Supplement

SELF DEFENSE
The Problem
The Solution
Weapons
Two Ways to Maim With A Crutch
Diversions
Home Protection
Dealing With the Neighbors' Dog
Group Tactics

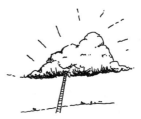

SHOPLIFTING FOR BEGINNERS

In view of today's economy, shoplifting should be thought of as a self-help program designed to give Senior Citizens a practical alternative to starving.
But there are rules ...

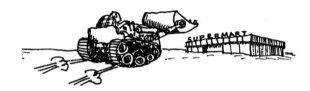

Basic Rules

DON'T FEEL GUILTY

If you're going to feel guilty, you might as well skip this section and go straight to Creative Cooking With Pet Foods.

DON'T BE GREEDY

Be selective. Use this practical survival skill to supplement basics like bread and water with prohibitively expensive luxuries like meat, cheese, butter, coffee, soap and laxatives.

DON'T BE OBVIOUS

Try not to draw attention to yourself. Better yet, work in pairs and get your confederate to create a timely diversion while you hobble into action.

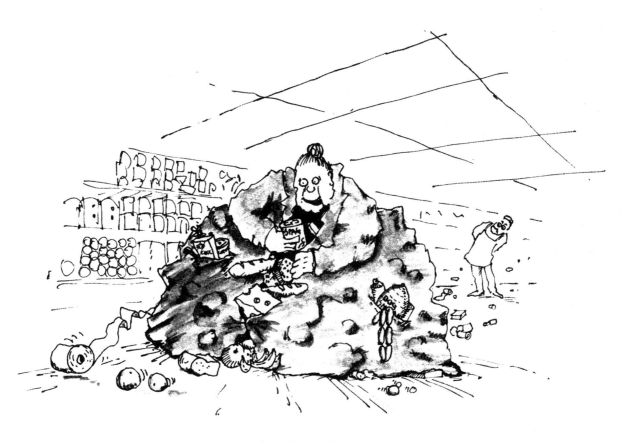

don't be greedy

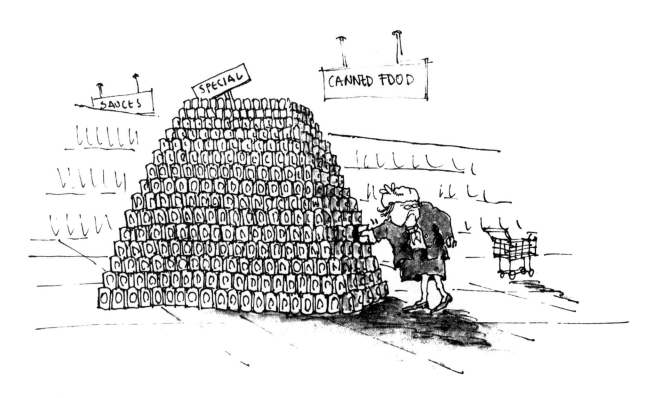

don't be obvious

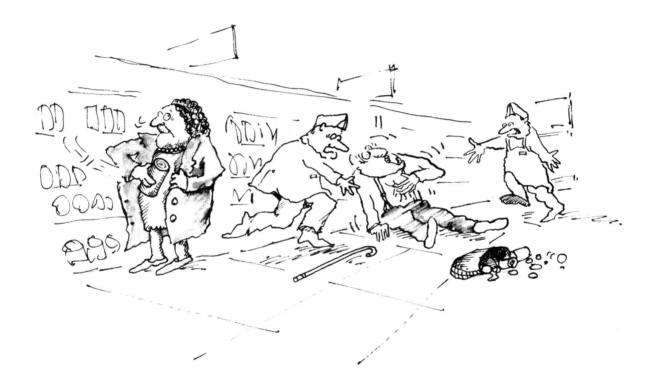

create a timely diversion

We Recommend ...

THE CHILD IN STROLLER RUSE

Borrow a child who's still young enough to burble incoherently. Borrow a stroller to put it in. If you can get paid for baby-sitting at the same time, so much the better!

Grab one of those hand-held shopping baskets on the way into the supermarket and fill it with unwanted basics while stuffing expensive luxury items underneath the child.

As you approach the checkout counter, casually lean down to the child and firmly pinch one of its pudgy little thighs. Use a hat pin if you prefer.

Appear concerned but helpless as the child erupts into a mega-decibel rage which drives everyone within hearing distance BONKERS.

Should the child show any sign of calming down, pinch, tweak or stick it again, so that it is screaming bloody murder by the time you reach the checkout.

Apologize profusely to the checker, dump your basket of basics on the counter and head quickly for the nearest exit.

Everyone will be so delighted to see both of you leave that no one will ever think to search the stroller.

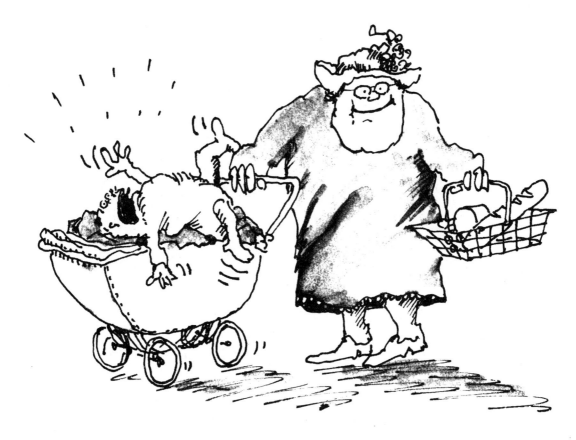

appear confused but helpless

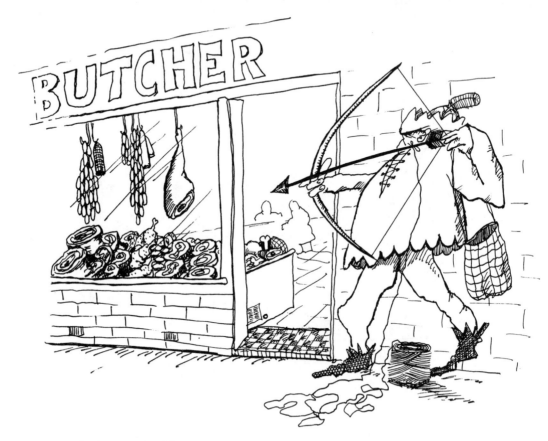

look upon shoplifting as an adventure, and remember Robin Hood

CREATIVE COOKING WITH PET FOODS

You have probably noticed that pet foods are really catching on with Senior Citizens these days.

Why?

Why not! Pet foods are packed with protein and are a great source of fiber. They are convenient, versatile and easy to use.

So why waste them on pets?

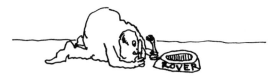

You Are What You Eat

Poverty aside, pet foods have become nutritionally superior to most people foods.
Compare the labels:
Why doesn't Chef Waldo tell you about vitamins, minerals, protein and calories?
What is Chef Waldo trying to hide?!?

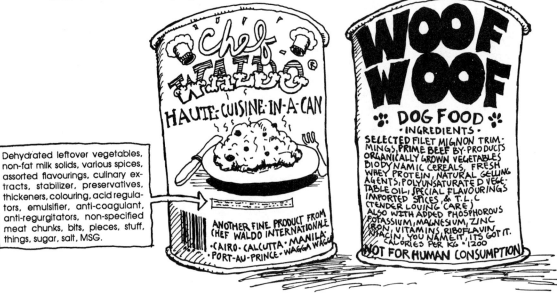

Dehydrated leftover vegetables, non-fat milk solids, various spices, assorted flavourings, culinary extracts, stabilizer, preservatives, thickeners, colouring, acid regulators, emulsifier, anti-coagulant, anti-regurgitators, non-specified meat chunks, bits, pieces, stuff, things, sugar, salt, MSG.

Chef WALDO ®
HAUTE·CUISINE·IN·A·CAN

ANOTHER FINE PRODUCT FROM CHEF WALDO INTERNATIONALE
·CAIRO· CALCUTTA· MANILA·
·PORT-AU-PRINCE· WAGGA WAGGA·

WOOF WOOF
❀ DOG FOOD ❀
·INGREDIENTS·
SELECTED FILET MIGNON TRIMMINGS, PRIME BEEF BY-PRODUCTS ORGANICALLY GROWN VEGETABLES BIODYNAMIC CEREALS, FRESH WHEY PROTEIN, NATURAL GELLING AGENTS, POLYUNSATURATED VEGETABLE OIL, SPECIAL FLAVOURINGS IMPORTED SPICES & T.L.C (TENDER LOVING CARE) ALSO WITH ADDED PHOSPHOROUS POTASSIUM, MAGNESIUM, ZINC IRON, VITAMINS, RIBOFLAVIN NIACIN, YOU NAME IT, ITS GOT IT. CALORIES PER KG ·1200
NOT FOR HUMAN CONSUMPTION

which would YOU rather eat?

Memorable Meals

Combine your favorite recipes with a variety of pet foods to create a series of memorable meals in a jiffy. Replace outrageously expensive meat and fish with wholesome, valued packed pet foods today!

Our chef suggests ...

HEALTHY BREAKFASTS
  Doggie Biscuits & Laying Mash Muesli
  Puppy-King Granola

LIGHT LUNCHES
  Go-Cat Tuna Salad
  Jellymeat Mousse
  Pal Liver Pâté
  Rabbit Mix Rissoles (vegetarian)
  Gourmet Pet Roll Pâté
  Chum Croquettes Rolled in
    Billy Peach Silver Sand

HEARTY MAINS
  Fido Meat Loaf
  Gravy Train Goulash
  Kitty Duck & Turkey Tureen
  Meaty Bites Stew
  Ruff-Ruff Beef & Pasta Casserole

SUCCULENT SEAFOOD
  Meow Bouillabaisse
  Biscat Bisque
  Sardines in Aspic on Toast

ETHNIC DELIGHTS
  Mexican: Chilli Con Kiblex
  American: Fidoburgers; Tuxettes Texas Style
  Chinese: Sweet 'n' Sour Jellychicken,
    Jellyfish & Cashews
  Japanese: Meow Sardine Sushi

DELICIOUS DESSERTS
  Doggie Bon-Bons & Ice Cream
  Budgie Seed Balls in Chocolate Sauce

Sample Recipe

MEAT LOAF AU FIDO
The beauty of cooking with pet foods is that most of the ingredients are already included.

For this moist and meaty Loaf, all you need is:
three large cans of Fido dog food
one large onion
one tbs. cooking oil
three pinches of salt
one large frying pan
a deep, loaf-shaped 'non-stick' baking pan

1) Open Fido cans
2) Gently sauté onion in well oiled frying pan
3) Stir in the Fido
4) Chuck the whole lot into the baking pan
5) Place in pre-heated oven on medium for 10 minutes.

Serves 4 adults, 6 weight-watchers or 1 teenager.

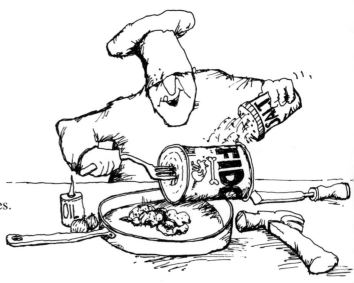

gently sautéed to perfection

Entertaining for the Impoverished

If the high cost of entertaining is all that's keeping you from throwing a gala dinner party, then have a look at this.

Apéritif – *'Attila'* After Shave (You can find countless unused bottles of this uniquely aromatic fluid at the local rubbish dump shortly after Fathers' Day).

Main Course – Assorted vegetables, (freshly selected from your grocer's rubbish) and Garfield Creme of Chicken on Rice (Shoplifted).

House Wine – Raspberry Kool-Aid in rubbing alcohol.

Dessert – Ten milligram tabs of Valium, suspended in Lime jello and eaten with chopsticks.

NOTE:

Should a meatier main course be desired, get in the habit of setting traps for small animals or neighborhood pets. (See *'How to Trap Neighbourhood Pets for Fun & Profit'*.)

STAYING HEALTHY
WHILE YOU'RE FALLING APART

Let's face it. If people were meant to live forever, they wouldn't start falling apart so soon. The best we can do is enjoy what we've got while it still works, and try not to do anything to encourage the process.

Of course, staying healthy helps. But not everybody is up to the task – especially if it means living your twilight years like a twelfth century Monk on a treadmill.

So what are the options? Well, some experts think we can stay healthy by watching our diets. Others think exercise is the answer.
A few actually recommend sex.

Our panel of unemployed experts recommends all three, plus two of these survival hints with a glass of water before bed.

DIET

Who says you can't have your cake and eat it too?

The only problem is that no one knows what it means.

According to our panel of experts, you should eat anything you want, whenever you want - and if it kills you, at least you won't die hungry.

EXERCISE

It's a well known fact. Exercise kills more Senior Citizens than streetcars. So be careful, do 'everything in moderation' and follow these recommendations:

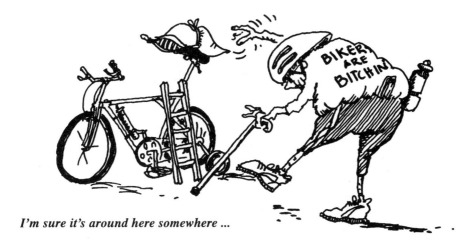

I'm sure it's around here somewhere ...

1. Bicycles may be fun, but think of how silly you look in lycra and a helmet.

2. Never engage in an exercise that makes you sweat.
3. Avoid any exercise that makes you wobble
   (Remember – Junior Citizens jog. Senior Citizens *jiggle*).

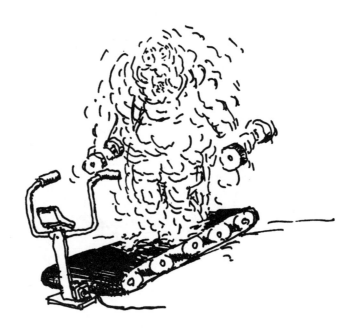

... please seek medical advice if jiggling persists over 5 minutes

SAFE SEX FOR SENIORS
Our panel of experts wouldn't want to suggest that sex is bad for geriatrics. However, please make sure your health insurance is up-to-date before you have a go at it. (Readers who turned to this section first should seek professional counseling as soon as possible.)

PERSONAL SPA BATH
Relaxation is considered to be one of life's great elixirs. So feel free to try this inexpensive and effective method after a long day watching soap operas.

Drop two tablets of Alka-Seltzer down the front of your underpants and jump into a bathtub full of hot water. (Not recommended for pacemaker users or people who turned to the previous section first.)

GLAMOUR HINTS FOR GERIATRICS

Growing old feels bad enough without having to look the part as
well. But thanks to modern cosmetic surgery, you can fold back
the years, tuck away the ravages of time, and look young
again.
At least from the neck up!

Do-It-Yourself Face Lifts
Unfortunately cosmetic surgery has become so
expensive that Senior Citizens are resorting to
do-it-yourself face lifting.
Despite obvious drawbacks, all you need
are some helping hands, a firm grip and a
lot of imagination – especially when you
check out the results in the mirror.

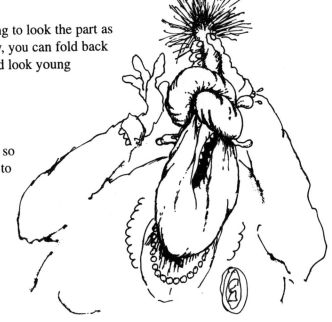

*gently pull loose skin up to top of head and secure in place,
camouflage with large hat, wig or well-gelled mohawk haircut*

don't worry if your body doesn't match your new face, people will think you're another rich American off a cruise ship

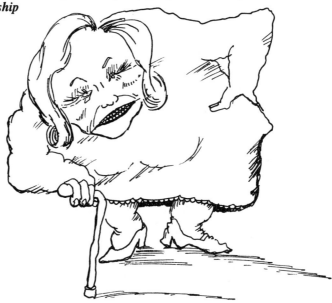

Staying in Style

Just because you are old and impoverished doesn't mean you can't dress in style. Maybe not this year's style. Maybe not even last year's style. But at least in some year's style!

So check out your local second-hand clothing shop. After all, the clothes you gave away to charity twenty years ago are probably this season's *haute couture*.

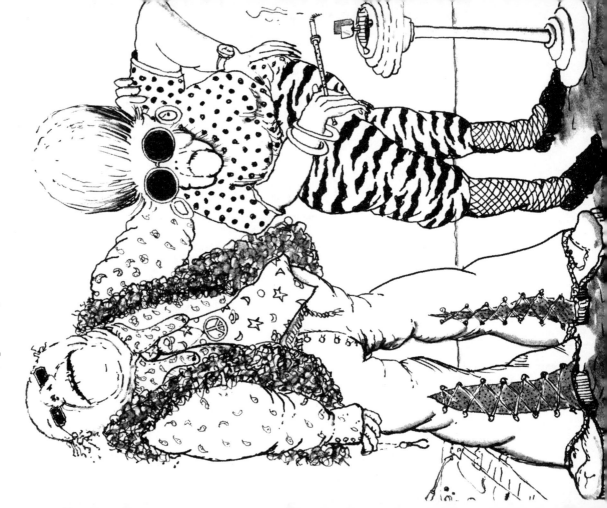

SALVATION ARMY FASHION SUPPLEMENT
CAUTION - HERNIA WARNING:
*Do not attempt to pull out without a trained nurse
or personal fitness consultant in attendance!*

SELF-DEFENSE

The Problem

Being a Senior Citizen these days is worse than being on the 'Endangered Species' list. Not only do you stand a good chance of being mugged, burgled or purse-snatched, you're fair game for every human parasite from con men to tax men.

Sad to say, today's society dismisses Senior Citizens as an obsolete minority group not worth protecting. Worse, they see you as a hopeless group of decaying old has-beens on automatic self-destruct (see glossary for more 'insulting terms').

The Solution

FIGHT BACK!!!

So what if you're a bit rusty and worn out. So what if you can't fight with your fists. You're still a long way from that doddering, moth-eaten old fossil they think you are (for even more insulting terms try the same glossary).

Even if you can't outrun 'em, you can outsmart 'em. Besides, who would expect a helpless, crumbling old relic like you to employ sophisticated self-defense techniques like these?

Weapons

CANES AND SWORD STICKS

The trouble with these 'traditional' weapons is that bludgeoning takes too much energy and punctured arteries are *so* messy. Besides, unless you are absolutely sure the first blow will permanently disable your attacker, it just might turn around and use your weapon on you.

UMBRELLAS

The metal tips on some models can be sharpened to a lethal point, and an automatic umbrella shoved firmly down an assailant's throat and triggered is known to cause extreme discomfort.

CAMERA FLASH

A small pocket camera with a built-in flash is perfect for causing temporary blindness, giving you the chance to apply your heavy, steel-capped walking shoes to the soft spots of your attacker's despicable little body. Remember – this was good enough for James Stewart in Hitchcock's classic, 'Rear Window.'

CAYENNE PEPPER

This versatile and exotic spice has so many interesting uses that we only have room to mention two. Fill an empty spray bottle with a well mixed solution of this fiery powder and ammonia or bleach. Spray directly in your assailant's eyes and continue on your way. If you are particularly annoyed with your attacker, you may reinforce your displeasure by dumping the unused contents of the cayenne container down its throat as you depart.

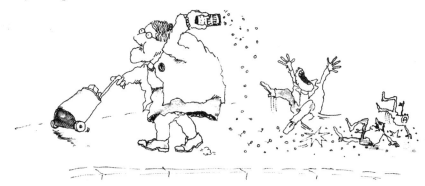

PILLS

When the odds are stacked against you and you have to run away, this little trick can save your life.

Hobble as far ahead of your pursuers as possible and spill your bottle of pills directly in their path.

They'll either slip on them and fall down – hopefully injuring themselves in the process – or they'll give up the chase in disgust at this pitiful gesture of defense.

NOTE: Don't use the last of your heart pills for this!

Two Ways to Maim with a Crutch
Killing with a crutch is easy. It's maiming that takes skill.

CAUTION; DO NOT ATTEMPT THESE TECHNIQUES ON STAIRS, MOVING ESCALATORS, WAXED FLOORS ... OR IF YOU NEED BOTH CRUTCHES TO REMAIN UPRIGHT.

THE ONE-CRUTCH CROTCH CRUNCHER
Wait until your assailant is within striking distance. Then suddenly look beyond it so that it thinks someone is coming up from behind.
As it turns to look, bring the left crutch up between its legs with enough force to lift it to its toes. This will cause it great pain followed by intense agony.
Take advantage of this moment to smash it over the back of its head and limp away, fastish.

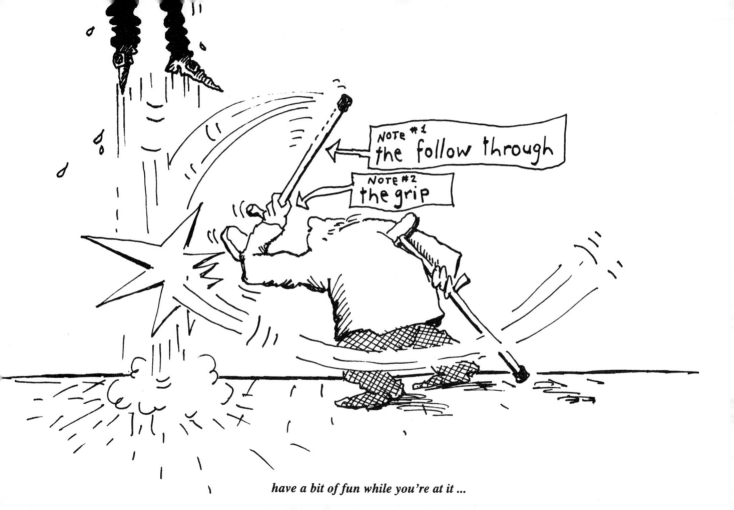

have a bit of fun while you're at it ...

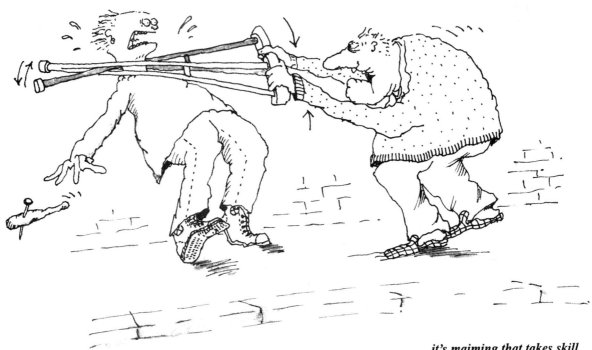

it's maiming that takes skill

THE TWO-CRUTCH PINCER
Judge your assailant's distance. Look it straight in the eye.
Aim for the neck. Thrust firmly with your right crutch. Follow through with your left,
and *squeeze* until the gutless little jerk loses consciousness.

Diversion

HIDE 'N' GO SEEK

For this little scam, you'll need mirrored sunglasses, steel-toed footwear, and a white lead-tipped cane.

Assuming that you are easy pickings, the cowardly muggers will approach more openly as you shuffle and tap your way through the rougher parts of town.

Using your cane 'feel' your way towards these worthless degenerates, tap around their feet. Stop, and say in a quavering voice, "Is anybody there?"

This will appeal to the muggers' perverted sense of humour, and give you the chance to kick one with your steel-toed carpet slipper while clobbering the other with your lead-weighted cane.

As they struggle to come to terms with this unexpected turn of events, remember that this trick will only work once, so quickly decide which parts of their bodies to damage more permanently.

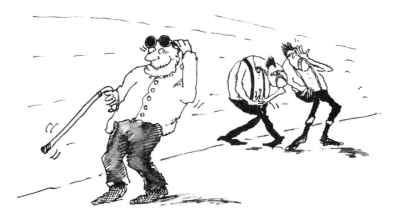

"Is anybody there?"

SHAKE-RATTLE-AND-ROLL

As a delaying tactic, this technique requires more co-ordination than acting skill, and can be very useful in a one-to-one confrontation.

First, make sure you are carrying a sock filled with sand and a pocket or coin-purse full of loose change.

When accosted and asked for money, start trembling (the more dramatic the better) and shakily fish out a handful of change.

Timidly offer it to your attacker with a sudden shudder so it tumbles to the ground at its miserable feet (if you need any motivation, just think of what might happen if this trick *doesn't* work)

As your over-confident assailant bends down to pick up its ill-gotten goods, whip out the sock full of sand and put it away.

Home Protection

GRANDCHILDREN, THE USE OF

When it comes to laying booby-traps, grandchildren are indispensable.

Pick the room where a burglar would most likely enter your home. Make sure you have plenty of toys, marbles, roller skates, and buiding-blocks on hand. Invite your grandchildren or neighbor's children over to play. You can throw them out after half an hour, that will be enough. Then close up the room and never invite them back. Any burglar entering this room is history.

SPRAY PAINT

The perfect weapon to use on obnoxious children and graffiti vandals. Always remember to shake the can before opening the door or sneaking up on the nasty vandals from behind.

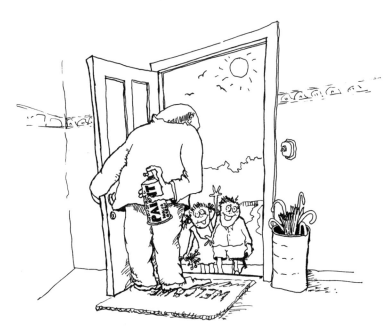

Hi Mr Jones, it's us again ...

NEIGHBORS' DOGS

It's a funny thing about neighbor's dogs. Their owners never seem to hear them bark or notice the daily deposits of recycled dog food their little darlings dump on other people's lawns. It's really not the dog's fault so let's deal with the inconsiderate clodheads who *are* responsible.

Tape record the sound of your neighbor's dog barking. That may mean getting up in the middle of the night or at the crack of dawn, but it will be worth it. Procure a large outdoor public address system and conceal the speaker or speakers near your neighbor's bedroom. If you can't get that close, just increase the volume. Connect to an electronic multi-timer set for 1:00am, 2:10am, 3:45am and 4:30am. Plug in your tape recorder, insert a pair of ear plugs and go to bed. Guaranteed to work.

For the other problem, simply scoop up the offending material as usual. Only this time, place the entire lot in your neighbor's letterbox, the driver's seat of their car or directly in front of their entry door before ringing the bell. Don't hang around.

... don't hang around.

FEAR

Why use a traditional security system that sounds an alarm which everyone, including the police, ignores. Install a device that plays a pre-recorded message like this:

> *"Welcome to the home of Don 'Vicious' Vicente, recently retired Godfather of the local Family. Don Vicente is sorry he has missed you, but is visiting the surviving relatives of the last person who entered his home without permission.*
> *Please do not bother to leave a message as hidden cameras have already recorded your identity. Have a nice day."*

Group Tactics

We know that Gangs are just groups of individual cowards who band together to make themselves feel brave. Why not use the same strategy to confront the enemy on its home turf.

Send out a suitable decoy to lull these brain-dead dorks into a false sense of security, then ...

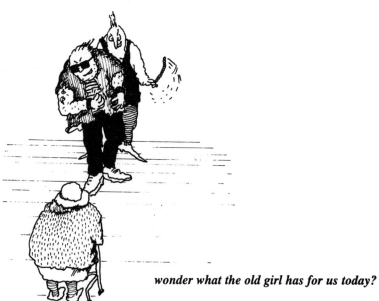

wonder what the old girl has for us today?

... **spring a trap that will make Custer's Last Stand look like a tea party!**

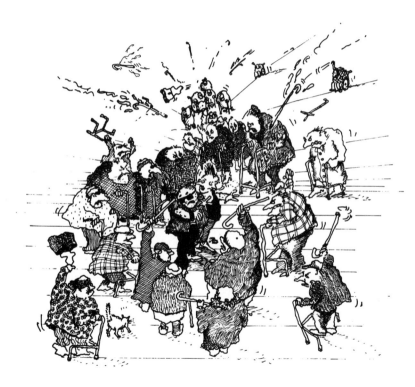

I want my MOMMMY!!!

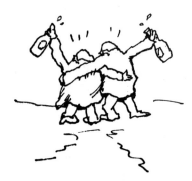

PART III - SOCIAL SKILLS

GROWING OLD *DIS*GRACEFULLY
Introduction
Toy Boys
Making the Most of Your Toy Boy

REVENGE, SWEET REVENGE
Introduction
Annoying Your Children
Embarrassing Them
Worrying Them
Making Them Feel Guilty
Driving Them Crazy

OUT TO PASTURE
Introduction
The Right Spot
Combating Boredom
Combating 'User Pays'

SENILITY AS A CON
Shopping
Public Transport
Eating Out

SOME ADVANTAGES OF BEING OLD
Advantages
Dealing with Religious Zealots

NEW PRODUCTS FOR OLD FOGIES
Introduction
Combination Microwave/TV
Swiss Army Hat
The Ezyboy Fart Converter
Electronic Toilet Paper Dispenser
Cooking with Chemicals Cookbook
How to Trap Neighborhood Pets for Fun & Profit
The Miracle TV Commercial Zapper

THE LAST LAUGH
Introduction
Adventures in Euthanasia
Cremations - Going Out With A Bang
High-flying Departures
Creative Thinking
The Last Word
On the Cheap
Over The Top
Where There's A Will ...
Glossary of Insulting Terms

Developing from a basic survivor into a sophisticated, finely-honey Social Activist is worth the effort, because it gives you a new lease on life.

Suddenly, shackles fall and the load finally lifts from shoulders too long stooped. Eyes brighten, sinews firm. The step quickens and blood, until recently coagulated in horrid little lumps like poorly-mixed custard, once again flows freely through your veins.

But there are tests ahead! Here's how to cope.

GROWING OLD *DIS*GRACEFULLY

As one of the 19th century's most elegant experts on the subject, Oscar Fingall O'Flahertie Willis Wilde wrote: *'One should never make one's début with a scandal. One should reserve that to give an interest to one's old age.'*

He was right, of course, but then Oscar was never a chap to follow his own advice. Alas, his tragically short, yet prolific life was something of a never ending scandal and he paid dearly for the privilege of being a splendidly outrageous eccentric during one of the most hypocritical periods of English history.

If anything, Oscar should have paid heed to this little gem, *'Beware of those who cut off others heads to make themselves look taller.'* If he had then perhaps the 6 foot 6 inch genius might have lived to show us what even greater scandal he was capable of.

So why should we fight the system instead of settling 'gracefully' in to a more traditional and socially accepted mode? Because ... it's *more fun*.

Toy Boys

It is one of the anomalies of 20th Century hypocrisy that when an older woman sets up house with a handsome, virile young man, she is considered to have got herself a 'toy boy.' On the other hand, when an older man takes up with a winsome, sexy young lass, it is most unlikely that she will be referred to as his 'toy girl' – even if the man is a decrepit old wreck (see glossary).

Don't let that bother you for one moment, ladies! March proudly into the new Millennium with your heads held high and the latest toy boy on your arm. After all, where would scandal be without hypocrisy?

Making the Most of Your Toy Boy

Having a toy boy around the house is only half the fun. You need to flaunt him in public to totally savor the brouhaha you have created.

DRESS HIM UP

Once you are committed to this course of action you might as well follow through. Dress your toy boy as if he were the toy girl of an aging big city car dealer. Insist on him wearing clothes that show off every muscle, curve and bulge to maximum effect. You'll soon learn to tell the difference between genuine shock and pure envy.

OLDER & BOLDER

The trouble with gossips and critics is that they say all the good stuff when your back is turned. That means you have to be somewhat innovative in your approach to inciting a reaction you can enjoy. Try this. Turn up at least ten minutes late to your next meeting of Older & Bolder, Gray Power or similar group, with toy boy in tow. Make sure the person conducting the meeting sees you enter and the look on their face is guaranteed to make everyone else turn around.

sorry we're late everybody...

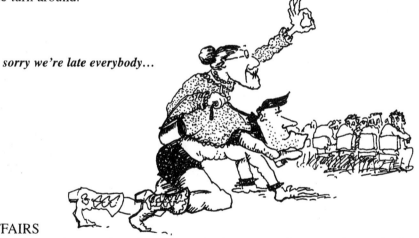

FAMILY AFFAIRS

For the ultimate in reactions, wait until a large gathering to reveal your toy boy to the family. Weddings, funerals, christenings and bar mitzvahs are best, but Christmas or Hanukkah will do in a pinch. Again– turn up at least ten minutes late. Once the initial shock dies down you can keep things stirred up by being overly affectionate, joking about your love life and mentioning your desire to appear on the Oprah Winfrey Show.

REVENGE, SWEET REVENGE

Whoever said that revenge isn't fun must have been a Junior Citizen. Besides, you may not get another chance.

Annoying Your Children
Annoying your offspring is easy - just do to them what they did to you while they were growing up.

PAY THEM A VISIT AND ...
• take along all your dirty washing.
• go straight to the refrigerator, carefully study the contents, complain that there's nothing you like, then devour everything in sight.

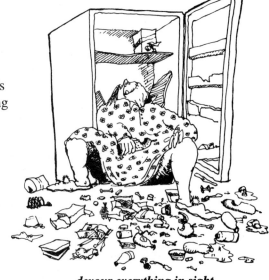

devour everything in sight

- leave a mess in every room and be sure to turn on all the lights.
- tie up their telephone for hours, making long-distance calls wherever possible.
- break a few of their favorite glasses.
- get up early and use up all the milk/coffee/tea, etc.
- switch on the TV then leave the room.
- crank up the volume on their stereo and insist you're hard of hearing when they ask you to turn it down.
- become suddenly infirm when asked to do anything to help around the house, then complain that you are bored.
- borrow their car and return it with a near-empty fuel tank.
- come home without it and say that you can't remember where you left it.
- come for a week ... stay for eight ... and pay for nothing.
- slam the door when you leave.

THE GOLDEN RULES
- borrow money, tools, clothes, etc, and never return them.
- call them collect from faraway places and ask them to send you the fare home.
- forget all their birthdays.
- phone them early Sunday morning, during dinner or in the middle of their favorite TV show and say you feel lonely and just thought you'd have a little chat.
- encourage your grandchildren to do all the rotten things their parents did at their age.
- never miss a chance to tell them that they just don't understand what it's like to be your age.

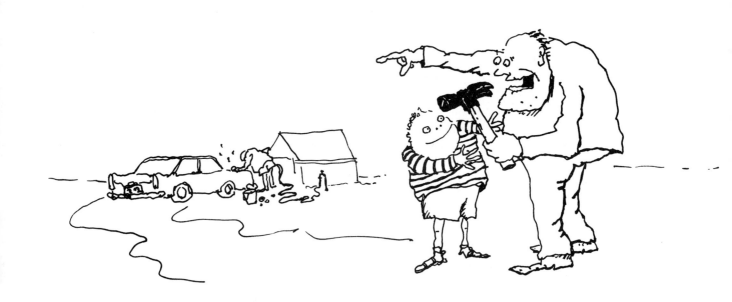

encourage your grandchildren to do what their parents did ...

Embarrassing Them

- dress in your best clothes and turn up at a particularly deserving offspring's place of work when you are sure they're away. Proudly tell everyone in sight that it's your birthday and you are being taken out for a special lunch. When someone explains that your offspring isn't there, say, "Oh ... guess they've forgotten again ..." and shuffle sadly away.
- dance at their wedding.
- surprise them at their next pool or spa party by jumping in nude.

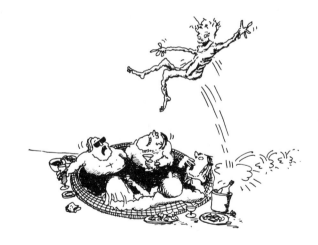

... surprise!!!

Or show up at their next important dinner party dressed in your grubbiest clothes and beg for food.

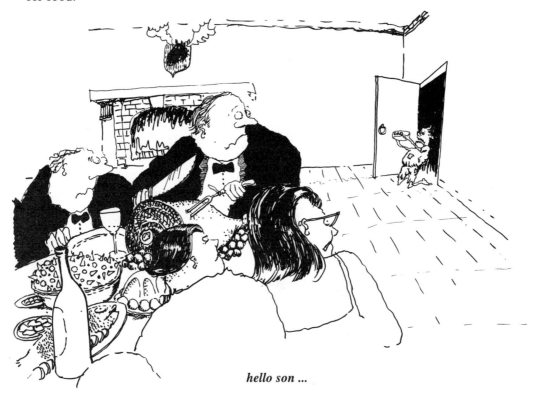

hello son ...

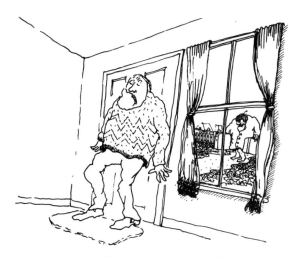

spending our last days with you....

Worrying Them

Should you have any second thoughts about worrying your children, simply cast your mind back to those sleepless nights, missed meals and gray hairs. Here are a few useful phrases:

I've been thinking ... it's about time I got married again.

Then once I've got my flying license I could buy a nice little plane.

Of course I know that Reverend Bobby has been indicted, it's just that he's so cute on TV.

Our agent says there are some great deals on package tours of Afghanistan, Iran, Somalia and Haiti right now.

What would you say about me joining one of those communes?

We've always counted on spending our last days with you.

Wonder how much money we could spend before we die ... ?

It's not too late to change my will you know!

And if none of the above works, take off on a two week vacation and forget to tell them.

Making Them Feel Guilty

Parents have been making their children feel guilty since the beginning of time. So why stop a good thing now? Here are some more useful phrases:

You wouldn't dare say that if your father was still alive.

Your mother would turn in her grave if she heard you speaking to me like that.

If only your father could hear you now.

And after all I've sacrificed for YOU!

Don't worry about me. You have your own life to live ... (accompanied by a sigh).

Guess I'm just no good for anything any more.

You won't have me to push around much longer.

I could just shrivel up and die for all you care.

You'll miss me when I'm gone.

At least my cat loves me.

Driving Them Crazy

When offspring visit you, or vice-versa, insist on taking them everywhere in your car. If they demur, you are totally justified in making them feel so guilty that they acquiesce meekly.

MAGIC MYSTERY TOUR

Let's say you're heading for the nearest shopping center. Who says you can't make a few un-scheduled stops along the way? And what's keeping you from pretending to get lost a few times - especially in the seedier sections of town? Remember, you were driving before they were born. So you have every right to change the rules as you go along.

JOURNEY FROM HELL

Give them a dose of their own medicine. At the first set of stop-lights challenge the car next to you to a drag race. Make sure to burn some rubber when the light changes, zig-zagging through traffic while using your horn and flipping the finger to anyone who gets in your way. Lurch in to a busy parking lot, whip in to the tightest space you can find and slam on your brakes. You'll enjoy the looks of sheer terror.

SLOW BOAT TO CHINA

Driving like a speed demon doesn't suit everyone. So here's a sure fire method that's been employed by Senior Citizens ever since the invention of the motor car. To really make sure this works you have to have a car that is capable of short bursts of speed.

If you can't find a two lane highway or popular country road, the far left lane of the freeway will suffice. Once you're in the traffic flow, gradually slow down to a speed well under the limit. Turn off your hearing aid so you're not distracted by the pleas of your offspring or the horns of the traffic building up behind. Avoid looking in the mirror and stay on the lookout for any opportunity for traffic to pass you. This is when a powerful engine will allow you to leave them in your dust until you can once again slow to a crawl.

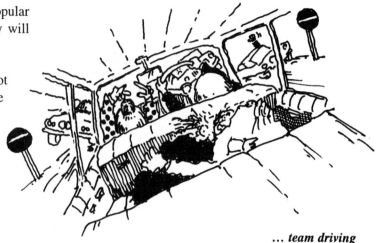

... team driving

TEAMWORK

Some couples find it best to drive as a team. This usually means that Dad operates the controls while Mom provides the instructions. If Mom can squeal, clutch the door, cover her eyes or stomp abruptly on an invisible brake peddle whenever another car comes close, so much the better. If you're on a country road with no other cars in sight Dad can turn to Mom and tell her an old joke. When someone in the back seat says, "Come on, Dad. There's a car coming ...", respond by turning around, looking your accuser straight in the eye and say, "So what?" Mom can liven things up even further by suddenly pointing at something in the distance and shouting, "My God. Look at that!!!" And if that doesn't seem to phase your offspring, try, "Did we tell you they canceled Dad's car insurance when he lost his license after that accident last year?"

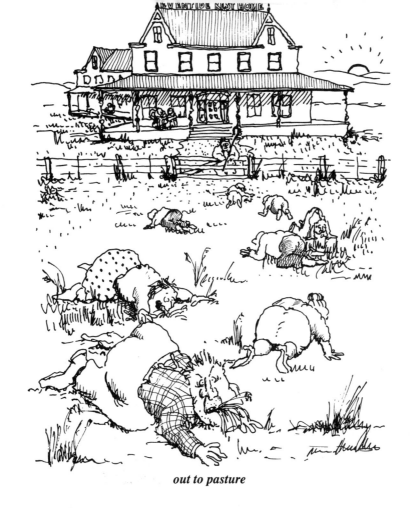

out to pasture

OUT TO PASTURE

In some societies, Senior Citizens are expected to spend the final years of their lives living in the comfort of the Family Home, surrounded by their children, grandchildren and great-grandchildren.

In others, old people are more or less expected to walk out into the wilderness to die alone.

With a choice like that it's no wonder that Retirement Communities are so popular.

Choosing The Right Spot

Whether it's a huge community of several thousand, a smaller, more intimate retirement village or an even smaller retirement home, it pays to check it out carefully before signing on the dotted line.

Here are some rules to follow.

Don't involve your children.
*They don't have to live there, but **you** do ...*

Pretend to be checking the place out for YOUR parents.
*Get an idea of what you can **really** expect.*

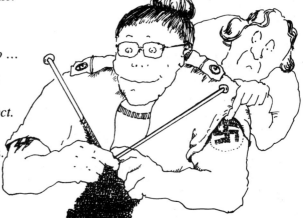

note: If you get a chance, check out the Matron's arms for suspicious tattoos.
You can never be too careful!

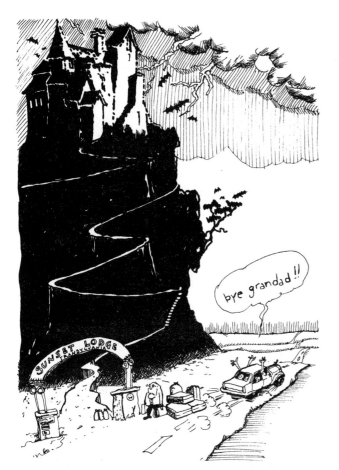

After the official tour, insist on a 'quiet hour' by yourself to 'get the feel of the place'. This gives you a chance to:

- cross-examine a few of the inmates.
- check the kitchen cupboards for large quantities of pet food.
- take a sample of the water for analysis (some places put embalming fluid in the drinking water to keep everyone looking younger).
- if possible, invite yourself to the next meal and insist on eating what the residents eat.
  compare this to what the staff eats and what the residents are paying for their food.
- inspect the records of the local ambulance service *be wary of an unusually high turnover.*

select your retirement spot carefully

Combating Boredom

OK. You've chosen your retirement spot and moved in. Now what?

Here are some suggestions to make sure that at least you're not bored to death:

• Home brewing is not only a fascinating hobby, it can help make you friends. Start with lagers and stouts, and graduate to your own still. Bathtub gin will ensure your popularity.
• Infiltrate the local Bridge Club and introduce a porn video night.
• Invite local Peeping Toms to start their own neighborhood-watch group.
• Organise practical adult education classes, like 'Do-It-Yourself Casket Making', 'Euthanasia For Beginners', or 'How to Con Welfare Agencies'.
• Sabotage the speed governors on the golf carts.

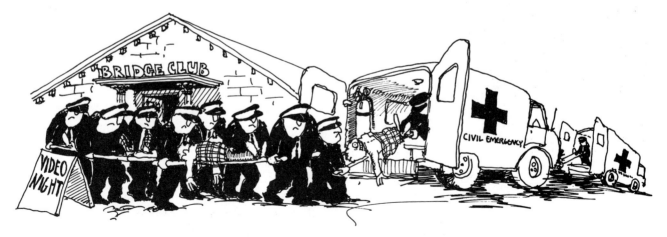

Combating 'User Pays'

If there was ever a term designed to put the wind up Senior Citizens, it's 'user pays'. Not only have succeeding Governments milked you for every spare cent throughout a lifetime of paying taxes, fees, licenses and duties – the shameless bloodsuckers now expect you – the 'client' – to continue paying for everything, including their inflated, undeserved pensions. Some ingenuity might help ease this insult to injury.

- Give everyone on a public hospital waiting list the 'opportunity' to go into a special weekly lottery. The winners get their operations straight away.
  Second prize is six months taken off the waiting time.
  Third prize gets to go ahead of the person in front.
  And if you get Fourth place you get a 10% discount on your funeral.
- Place slot machines in every drugstore. Win the Jackpot and get your heart pills for free.
- Send a bill to your children for all the time, effort and money you have spent on them during their lives.
- Send a bill to the Government, charging $10 for every time a politician has welched on an election promise. You could make a fortune.

SENILITY AS A CON

The nicest thing about taking advantage of your age is that you're only doing what young people expect, and therefore deserve.

Shopping
FASTER SHOPPING

Senior Citizens should not be expected to spend their Golden Years standing around in supermarkets waiting to be checked-out.

Go straight to the front of the line, barge-in, pretending you are deaf should anyone complain, or push your fully laden shopping cart up to the '10 items or less' Express counter, ignoring all the dirty looks.

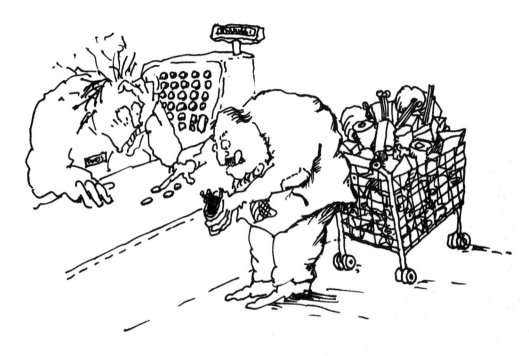

appear confused …

DISCOUNT SHOPPING

When asked to pay, appear confused when counting out your money and put down less than required.

When the checker points out your mistake, take back all the money and start again.

After a while the checker or another customer will pay the difference just to get rid of you.

Public Transport
FREE BUS RIDES

Push to the front of the line, using cane on shins where necessary. Get on first and stall the driver with small-talk and questions, while fumbling around pockets or purse in a futile search for money.

Continue this routine until the folks behind you start grumbling at the driver and someone – anyone – offers to pay your fare.

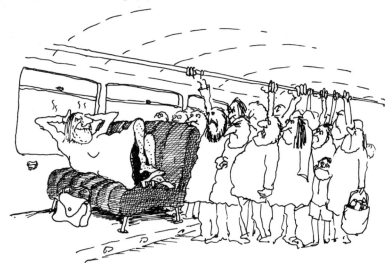

stretch out in comfort

NO STANDING

If all seats are occupied, limp painfully to the nearest Junior Citizen, demand its seat and wheeze directly into its face until it moves. When seated, start to tell the person next to you your life story, and soon you should be able to stretch out in comfort.

Eating Out
FREE LUNCH

Choose a decent restaurant. Enjoy an expensive meal. Walk out without paying.

If someone comes after you demanding payment, insist you've already paid ... you remember it clearly ... or at least you think you do ... but of course you do ... you've never forgotten before ... or at least you don't remember ever having forgotten before ... besides, here's the receipt (produce a bus ticket) ... who put that there? ... and so on ... Considering what it's costing for this person to listen to such drivel, there will eventually come a time when it becomes uneconomic and you're left to digest your meal in peace.

SOME ADVANTAGES OF BEING OLD

- Meals on Wheels ladies flirt with you.
- Buying a round of drinks down at the local tavern gets cheaper as your friends die off.
- You don't have to change your underwear so often.
- You can get away with driving your mobility cart like a lunatic.
- You can leave the toilet seat down more often.

Another advantage is that religious zealots don't try so hard to recruit you, although they are still happy to hit you up for donations.

Here are some tips on how to deal with these tedious hustlers:
- Ask for a receipt.
- Say you haven't seen their guru/leader since you served time together for fraud and are sorry to see that he/she still hasn't gone straight.
- If they're an eastern cult, invite them to your next Bible class.
- If they're 'bible bashers', invite them to a séance at the Theosophical Hall.
- If they try to get you to subscribe to a free monthly magazine, ask them how much money they'll pay you if you do.
- If they look like they've come straight off a farm in Utah and were brought up on dairy products, invite them in to look at your pornography collection.
- Otherwise, tell them to buzz off!

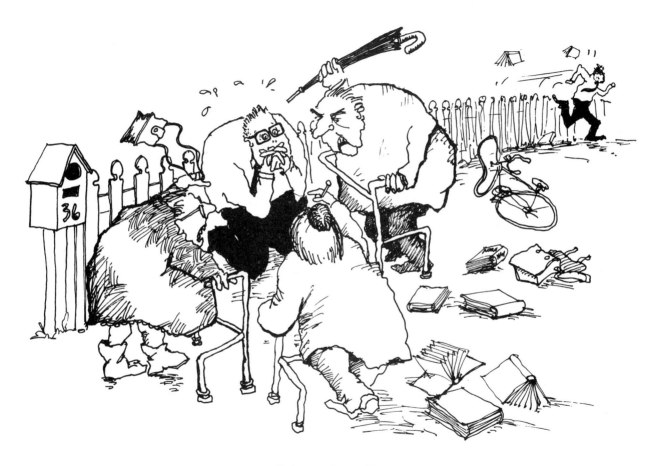

tell them to buzz off

NEW PRODUCTS FOR OLD FOGIES

What will technology offer Senior Citizens in the 21st Century? Will manufacturers finally recognize the need to cater for this rapidly growing consumer market?
I wouldn't hold your breath.

But here are just a few of the amazing inventions and practical new products that we can expect to see if they ever do.

Combination Microwave/TV
Say 'goodbye' to watching plucked fowls rotate slowly through small glass doors. With *MicroTele* you'll never again miss your favorite soap opera, talk show or infommercial while slaving over a cold microwave. New micro-screen technology transforms the ordinary microwave door into a TV screen - and your favorite TV stars into turkeys. Includes remote control and stereo speakers.

Swiss Army Hat
For the gadget conscious Senior Citizen who has everything.

The Ezyboy Fart Converter
Turn useless old farts into $$$. Cook, heat and run your TV on methane gas from your very own personal *Fart Converter* from *Ezyboy*. And with the simple addition of the optional *Ezyboy MegaMethane Booster*, you can even run your golf cart and lawn mower. All without leaving the comfort of your favorite easy chair.

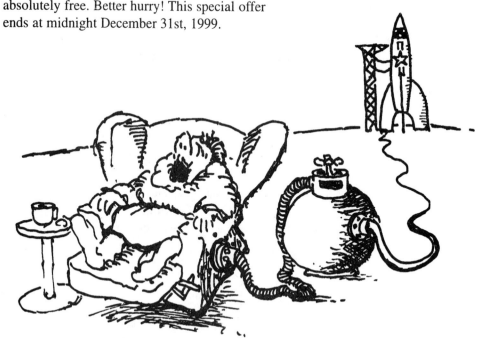

the Ezyboy Fart Converter ... but be quick, supplies are limited

Electronic Toilet Paper Dispenser

Let's face it! Everyone uses toilet paper. But do they have to use so much? Now you can control TP use with the revolutionary new ETPD. Perfect for guests and visiting relatives. You program the number of sheets. An electronic voice reminds each user of our dwindling rain forests and warns them how many segments they've got left. The automatic counter stops dispensing TP at the pre-programed number ... and you SAVE! Optional Coin or Credit Card activated models available. Perfect for retirement homes, accountants and millionaires.

Cooking With Chemicals Cookbook

Ideal for the supermarket shopper who reads all the food labels. Why pay some multinational food giant to manufacture your meals from unpronounceable ingredients? Learn to create unforgettable meals with your very own chemical cocktail. Index of long-term side effects not included.

How to Trap Neighbourhood Pets For Fun & Profit
An informative and useful 'how to' book that offers practical advice on how to increase your protein intake while earning extra money selling the surplus. Complete with instructions, three easy-to-use traps (small, medium and large) and preparation hints. See *Cooking with Pet Foods* for exciting recipe ideas.

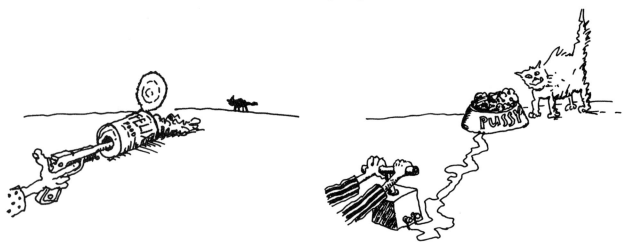

here Kitty-Kitty!

It's a *Miracle* TV Commercial *Zapper*

At last! Now you can protect your ears from those overly loud and patronising TV commercials with the astounding *Miracle Zapper*. Simply set your TV to a comfortable volume and enjoy your favorite show. When the commercials come on and start blaring away, the electronic wizardy of the *Miracle Zapper* will automatically activate the mute control until the volume returns to something reasonable.

THE LAST LAUGH

You may not be able to avoid the inevitable, but with a little forethought, a smidgen of imagination and a dollop of good old vindictive bile, you can make bloody sure that those you leave behind know damn well 'who got the last laugh'!

Adventures In Euthanasia
The euthanasia we're talking about shouldn't be confused with the teenage religious movement in Singapore.

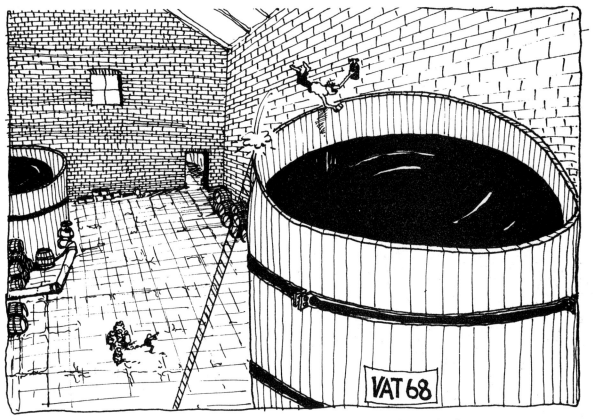

Arrange for a tour of your favorite Whisky distillery, and at the appropriate moment, execute a 'swan dive' into the vat of your choice. It should not be difficult to avoid rescuers.

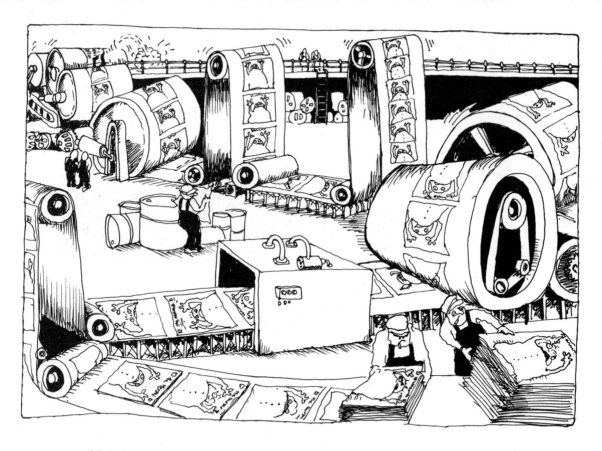

Visit the newspaper you love to hate. Wait until the final edition is rolling, then hurl yourself between the rollers – you really *will* make the front page!

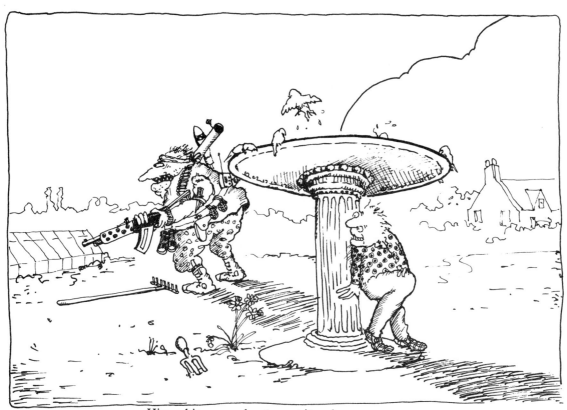

Hire a hitman and outsmart it as long as you can.

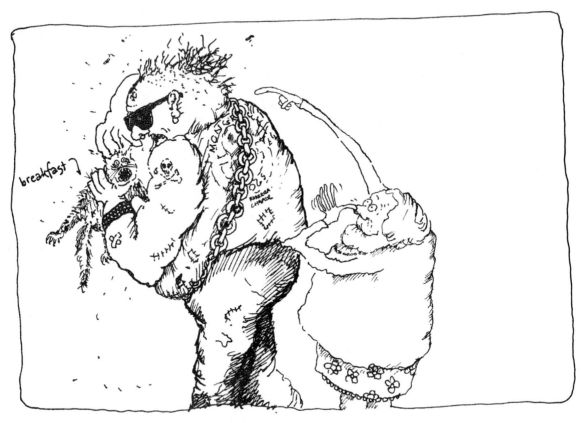

Tell a gang member just how silly it looks

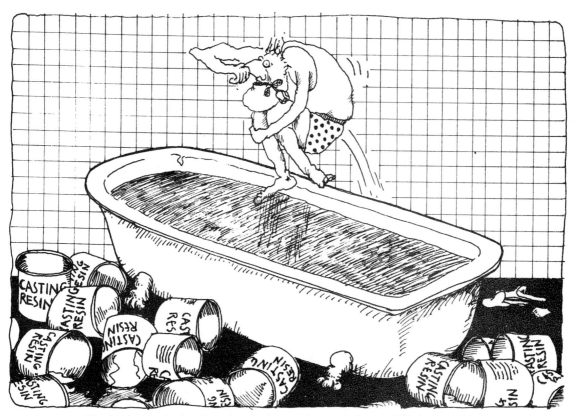

Expire into a bath of casting resin and become the world's largest door stop.

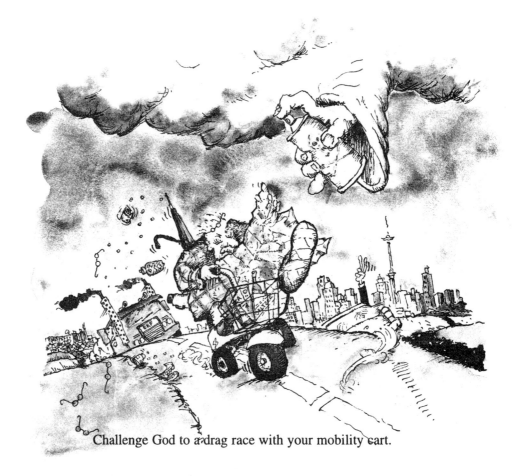

Challenge God to a drag race with your mobility cart.

Going Out with a Bang

With space at a premium these days, more and more people are opting for cremation. besides, it could be good practice for the next stop!

BIG BANG
By the time anyone finds out you've stuffed your homemade casket with high explosive, you'll be long gone.

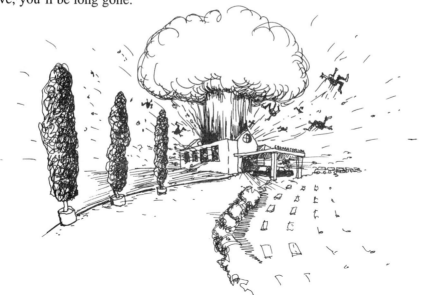

CHINESE NEW YEAR
How about a less expensive variation? Insist on being decked out in a favorite suit or dress, previously lined with firecrackers.

FRESH AIR FAREWELL (or *Hire-A-Pyre*)
For a funeral al fresco, line up a couple of old Army buddies who, at the appropriate moment, will step forward with flame-throwers and really see you out.

High Flying Departures
If cost is no problem – or if you want to leave behind as little as possible – hire a helicopter to deposit your remains at famous landmarks such as the torch on the Statue of Liberty, the top of the Eiffel Tower, the summit of your favorite mountain, the spire of a cathedral or the pinnacle of one of those obnoxious downtown towers that seem to be popping up all over the place like pimples on an adolescent's face.

Creative Thinking

Speaking of favorite spots, think about arranging for 'life's empty shell' to be permanently concealed close to somewhere special, like the green where you scored your first hole-in-one.

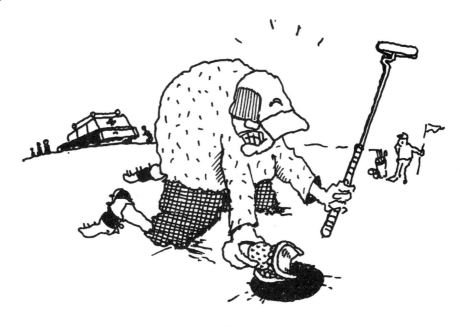

... your first hole in one

The Last Word

For the last word in burials, have a tape player secreted in your casket and get a friend **to** activate the remote control which activates your voice at the perfect moment ...

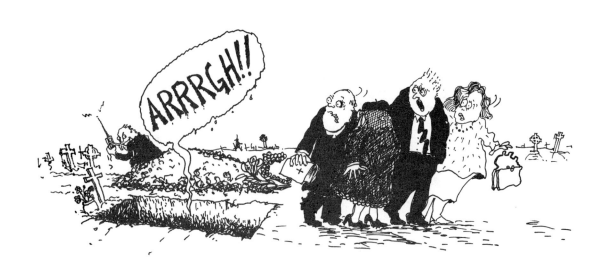

On The Cheap
Inexpensive burials don't necessarily mean a cardboard casket, especially with a little forward planning - and a little help from your friends.
• Have yourself packed and anonymously
shipped to the Welfare Department or IRS. COD!

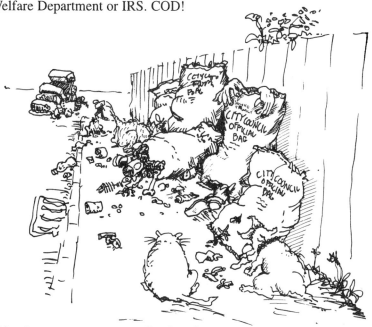

• Arrange for a friend to put you out on collection day.

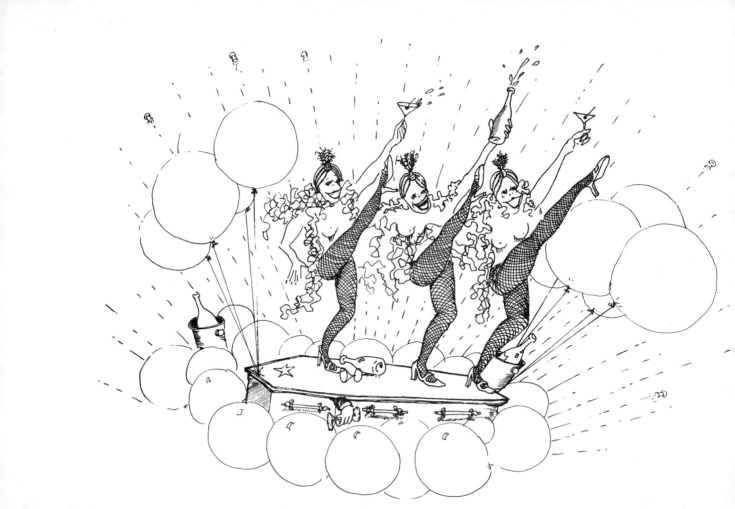

Over The Top
Cheap funerals might not suit every body, so here's an expensive but memorable alternative.

SHOW TIME
A Hollywood producer will need to work closely with an Archbishop on this extravaganza, as nothing less than a large cathedral will do.

After a suitably solemn intro by his Bishopness, exotically clad dancers from Las Vegas will perform a choreographed version of your life.
This will be followed with a selection of your favourite songs, sung by the Three Tenors, accompanied by the London Philharmonic Orchestra under the baton of John Williams, with solos from Jesse Norman and Paul McCartney.
The eulogy will be delivered – with appropriate pauses and meaningful looks – by Prince Charles of Britain, reading a script prepared by someone named Camilla.
Your lead-lined, gold and silver encrusted casket will be transported comfortably to its final resting place in a custom built Maserati hearse, and buried with full military honors by surviving members of Saddam Hussein's bodyguard.

Your children will be sent the bill.

Where There's a Will ...
This is definitely your last chance to hit 'em where it hurts.

Thanks to our near-inviolate legal system (made so through the dedicated avarice of lawyers) a properly attested Will is a thing of joy, a forever document.
Disputed over, argued about, killed for.
It is not only your Last Testament – it is your Last Test of Them!

Here are a few suggestions:
• leave everything to the Dallas Cowboys Cheerleaders' Retirement Fund
• or to the Arnold Schwarzenegger For President Fund.
• or to the Timothy Leary Home for the Self Embalmed.
• or stick a pin in the Inner Mongolian telephone directory.
• or leave little treasure maps for everyone, with riddles for them to solve before they can hope to find the loot you've hidden away over the years.
• **But don't forget to leave a copy of this book to each of your children. One day they will need it too.**

A WILL WITH A TWIST

Now that you've been laid to rest as per your wishes, you might as well have one more Last Laugh.

To ensure a large gathering of family, friends, business associates, neighbors, etc, instruct your lawyers to invite everyone you've ever known to a large hall for the reading of your Will - suggesting they might learn 'something to their advantage'.

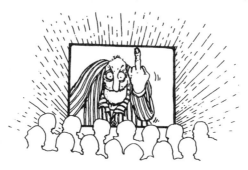

When they are all seated quietly, your lawyer will invite each guest to get up and say a few nice words about you. Each will be given a copy of a video you recorded before your demise, while the original is played on a large screen. This is your last chance to say all of the things you've ever wanted to say to various individuals in the audience; recommend that they enjoy the party afterwards, because all of your money went to pay for it.

GLOSSARY OF INSULTING TERMS

ancient old heap
at death's door
bag of old bones
blue-rinse brigade
bumbling old twit
cantankerous old coot
crumbling old relic
crusty old fart
decrepit old wreck
desiccated old pudwhipper
dim headed old dotard
dingey as a wooden watch
disagreeable old goat
doddering old twit
dried up old stump
falling apart at the seams
flatulent old frump
fuddy-duddy
fusty old fool

gone to seed
grizzled old curmudgeon
grubby old grump
grumpy old grub
had it
has-been
headed for the scrap heap
ineffectual old twerp
insignificant old dork
interfering old busy-body
lecherous old wobble-guts
living on borrowed time
long-in-the-tooth
malicious old gob-wobbler
moth-eaten old windbag
moldy oldie
muddle-brained old wally
museum piece
nasty old hag

nasty old man
never been
no spring chicken
noddle-brained old flipgibbet
obnoxious old fart-knocker
obsolete old gunge-bag
obstreperous old grouch
old bag
old dweeb
old fogy
old fool
old fuss budget
old numb-nuts
old timer
old wanker
oldie but moldy
one foot in the grave
ornery old cuss
ossified old fossil
out of the Ark
over the hill
passé

past it
past your prime
pathetic old dimwit
persnickety old git
rancid old knobhead
rickety old geezer
rusty and dusty
sagging old slag
sanctimonious old lecher
shriveled-up old rag-bag
snoopy old snipe
silly old ding bat
stale as an old ashtray
stubborn old mule
supercilious old sow
tiresome old geek
toothless old relic
walking worm fodder
way past it
whining old grumble-guts
worn out old crank
worthless old wrinkly

TITLES BY CCC PUBLICATIONS

Blank Books ($3.99)
SEX AFTER BABY
SEX AFTER 30
SEX AFTER 40
SEX AFTER 50

Retail $4.95 – $4.99
"?" book
CAN SEX IMPROVE YOUR GOLF?
THE COMPLETE BOOGER BOOK
FLYING FUNNIES
MARITAL BLISS & OXYMORONS
THE ADULT DOT-TO-DOT BOOK
THE DEFINITIVE FART BOOK
THE COMPLETE WIMP'S GUIDE TO SEX
THE CAT OWNER'S SHAPE UP MANUAL
THE OFFICE FROM HELL
FITNESS FANATICS
YOUNGER MEN ARE BETTER THAN RETIN-A
BUT OSSIFER, IT'S NOT MY FAULT
YOU KNOW YOU'RE AN OLD FART WHEN...
1001 WAYS TO PROCRASTINATE
HORMONES FROM HELL II
SHARING THE ROAD WITH IDIOTS
THE GREATEST ANSWERING MACHINE MESSAGES
WHAT DO WE DO NOW??
HOW TO TALK YOU WAY OUT OF A TRAFFIC TICKET
THE BOTTOM HALF
LIFE'S MOST EMBARRASSING MOMENTS
HOW TO ENTERTAIN PEOPLE YOU HATE
YOUR GUIDE TO CORPORATE SURVIVAL
NO HANG-UPS (Volumes I, II & III – $3.95 ea.)
TOTALLY OUTRAGEOUS BUMPER-SNICKERS ($2.95)

Retail $5.95
30 – DEAL WITH IT!
40 – DEAL WITH IT!

50 – DEAL WITH IT!
60 – DEAL WITH IT!
OVER THE HILL – DEAL WITH IT!
SLICK EXCUSES FOR STUPID SCREW-UPS
SINGLE WOMEN VS. MARRIED WOMEN
TAKE A WOMAN'S WORD FOR IT
SEXY CROSSWORD PUZZLES
SO, YOU'RE GETTING MARRIED
YOU KNOW HE'S A WOMANIZING SLIMEBALL WHEN...
GETTING OLD SUCKS
WHY GOD MAKES BALD GUYS
OH BABY!
PMS CRAZED: TOUCH ME AND I'LL KILL YOU!
WHY MEN ARE CLUELESS
THE BOOK OF WHITE TRASH
THE ART OF MOONING
GOLFAHOLICS
CRINKLED 'N' WRINKLED
SMART COMEBACKS FOR STUPID QUESTIONS
YIKES! IT'S ANOTHER BIRTHDAY
SEX IS A GAME
SEX AND YOUR STARS
SIGNS YOUR SEX LIFE IS DEAD
MALE BASHING: WOMEN'S FAVORITE PASTIME
THINGS YOU CAN DO WITH A USELESS MAN
MORE THINGS YOU CAN DO WITH A USELESS MAN
RETIREMENT: THE GET EVEN YEARS
LITTLE INSTRUCTION BOOK OF THE RICH & FAMOUS
WELCOME TO YOUR MIDLIFE CRISIS
GETTING EVEN WITH THE ANSWERING MACHINE
ARE YOU A SPORTS NUT?
MEN ARE PIGS / WOMEN ARE BITCHES
THE BETTER HALF
ARE WE DYSFUNCTIONAL YET?
TECHNOLOGY BYTES!
50 WAYS TO HUSTLE YOUR FRIENDS

HORMONES FROM HELL
HUSBANDS FROM HELL
KILLER BRAS & Other Hazards Of The 50's
IT'S BETTER TO BE OVER THE HILL THAN UNDER IT
HOW TO REALLY PARTY!!!
WORK SUCKS!
THE PEOPLE WATCHER'S FIELD GUIDE
THE ABSOLUTE LAST CHANCE DIET BOOK
THE UGLY TRUTH ABOUT MEN
NEVER A DULL CARD
THE LITTLE BOOK OF ROMANTIC LIES

Retail $6.95
CYBERGEEK IS CHIC
THE DIFFERENCE BETWEEN MEN AND WOMEN
GO TO HEALTH!
NOT TONIGHT, DEAR, I HAVE A COMPUTER!
THINGS YOU WILL NEVER HEAR THEM SAY
THE SENIOR CITIZENS'S SURVIVAL GUIDE
IT'S A MAD MAD MAD SPORTS WORLD
THE LITTLE BOOK OF CORPORATE LIES
RED HOT MONOGAMY
LOVE DAT CAT
HOW TO SURVIVE A JEWISH MOTHER

Retail $7.95
WHY MEN DON'T HAVE A CLUE
LADIES, START YOUR ENGINES!
ULI STEIN'S "ANIMAL LIFE"
ULI STEIN'S "I'VE GOT IT BUT IT'S JAMMED"
ULI STEIN'S "THAT SHOULD NEVER HAVE HAPPENED"

NO HANG-UPS – CASSETTES Retail $5.98
Vol. I: GENERAL MESSAGES (M or F)
Vol. II: BUSINESS MESSAGES (M or F)
Vol. III: 'R' RATED MESSAGES (M or F)
Vol. V: CELEBRI-TEASE